The ABC'S of Health and Wellness from A to Z

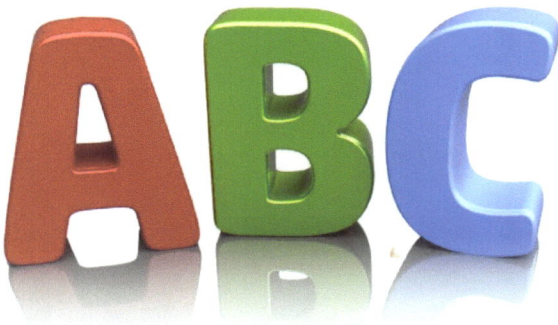

ABC

By ARIAN & MEGAN SMITH

Purpose Publishing
1503 Main Street #168 ♠ Grandview, Missouri
www.purposepublishing.com

ISBN: 978-0-9979853-0-6

Editing by Edna Williams Emerald Word Processing
emeraldwordp@gmail.com
Book Cover Design by PP Team of Designers

For permission and requests, write to the publisher:
1503 Main Street, #168, Grandview, MO 64030.

Author Inquiries may be sent
to contactus@purposepublishing.com

INTRODUCTION

As children, one of the first things you learn is the alphabet! It is the basic and beginning attribute of reading. Without the alphabet, it would be impossible to read. Am I right?!

Well just like your health there are beginning stages to developing and learning how to live a healthier lifestyle, as well. The ABCs of Health and Wellness is designed to introduce you to some healthier ideas in food, exercise and everyday living, one letter at a time.

Our goal is that living a healthier lifestyle will become easier and that the daily activities inside will aid in parent/child relationship building, teacher/student relationship building, and just all around team building!

First, let's take a look at a Sample Weekly Meal Planner, and then we'll dive into these ABCs...

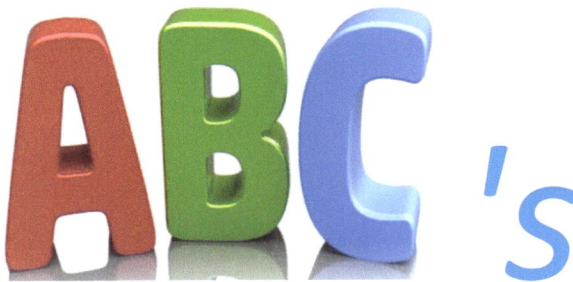

Day	Meal 1	Meal 2	Meal 3
Sunday	3 scrambled eggs ¼ cup of dry oatmeal Cup of orange, apple or grape	1 Apple or 1 medium banana, or 1 cup of sliced watermelon	4oz-6oz of chicken (baked or grilled) ½ cup of roasted red potatoes and 1 cup of green beans
Monday	3 scrambled eggs 2 slices of turkey bacon 2 slices whole grain toast	½ Grapefruit or 2 medium kiwi or ¾ cups of grapes	93%-96% lean ground beef w/ whole wheat tortilla, lettuce, light cheese & salsa (tacos)
Tuesday	¼ cup Whole grain cream of wheat ½ cup of berries	1 medium orange or 1 medium peach or 1 medium pear	4oz-6oz lemon pepper chicken ½ cup of steamed broccoli
Wednesday	3 scrambled eggs ¼ cup of oatmeal ½ sliced strawberries	8 medium strawberries or sliced pineapples or ½ cup of cherries	Spaghetti w/ whole grain pasta, 93%-96% lean ground beef or ground turkey & natural sauce
Thursday	¼ cup of Kix cereal or Special K with Almond Milk or Skim Milk	2 medium plums or 1 medium tangerine or ¼ medium cantaloupe	Tuna fish sandwich on 2 slices of whole grain bread w/ 2 medium celery sticks
Friday	¼ cup of Kix cereal or Special K with Almond Milk or Skim Milk	1 Apple or 1 medium banana or 1 medium peach	Sliced turkey on whole grain bread w/ baked chips & grape, apple or orange juice
Saturday	2 slices of pancakes 2 slices of turkey bacon 2 eggs scrambled	8 medium strawberries or sliced pineapples or ½ cup of cherries	Family Outing Enjoy It!

Sample Weekly Meal Planner

Meal 4	Meal 5	Notes
1 medium orange or 1 medium peach or 1 medium pear	4oz-6oz salmon 2 cups of broccoli	Snack Options: Fat free Greek yogurt, cottage cheese, low fat popcorn, rice cakes, granola bar or smoothie
8 medium strawberries or sliced pineapples or ½ cup of cherries	4oz-6oz tilapia (baked or grilled) w/ asparagus & sliced tomatoes	Snack Options: Fat free Greek yogurt, cottage cheese, low fat popcorn, rice cakes, granola bar or smoothie
1 Apple or 1 medium banana, or 1 cup of sliced watermelon	4oz-6oz chicken w/ stir fry veggies	Snack Options: Fat free Greek yogurt, cottage cheese, low fat popcorn, rice cakes, granola bar or smoothie
½ Grapefruit or 2 medium kiwi or ¾ cups of grapes	Chicken salad w/ sliced tomato, cucumbers and extra virgin olive oil or fat-free dressing	Snack Options: Fat free Greek yogurt, cottage cheese, low fat popcorn, rice cakes, granola bar or smoothie
8 medium strawberries or sliced pineapples or ½ cup of cherries	4oz-6oz tilapia (baked or grilled) w/ 1 cup of cooked kale	Snack Options: Fat free Greek yogurt, cottage cheese, low fat popcorn, rice cakes, granola bar or smoothie
½ Grapefruit or 2 medium kiwi or ¾ cups of grapes	Whole grain pizza crust w/ 93%-96% lean beef, veggies, light cheese & pizza marinara	Snack Options: Fat free Greek yogurt, cottage cheese, low fat popcorn, rice cakes, granola bar or smoothie
1 Apple or 1 medium banana or 1 medium peach	93%-96% lean ground beef or ground turkey & natural sauce w/ chili beans, stewed tomato & veggies(Pot of chili)	Snack Options: Fat free Greek yogurt, cottage cheese, low fat popcorn, rice cakes, granola bar or smoothie

GETTING STARTED

Nutrition

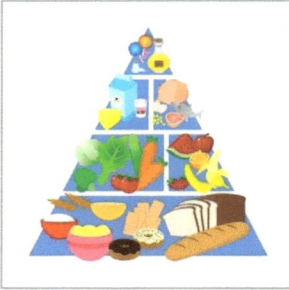

Nutrition is one of the most important things in our everyday life. Proper nutrition can prevent diseases, obesity and provide us with good energy.

Vitamins & Minerals

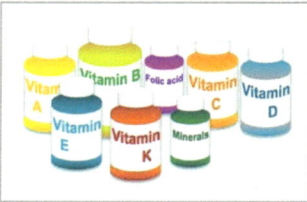

Often neglected, but also very important for our overall health are vitamins and minerals. There are so many added benefits when having them as a daily part of our lives.

Activities

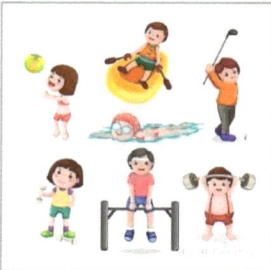

NO GYM? NO PROBLEM! There are many activities that can be done at home, in the backyard or at a park ~ activities that can be good and fun for everyone involved.

TABLE OF CONTENTS

Introduction.. 3
Meal Plans... 4
Getting Started... 6
Letter A 8
Letter B 9
Letter C 10
Letter D 11
Letter E 12
Letter F 13
Letter G 14
Letter H 15
Letter I 16
Letter J 17
Letter K 18
Letter L 19
Letter M 20
Letter N 21
Letter O 22
Letter P 23
Letter Q 24
Letter R 25
Letter S 26
Letter T 27
Letter U 28
Letter V 29
Letter W 30
Letter X 31
Letter Y 32
Letter Z 33
You Made It! 34
About the Authors 35

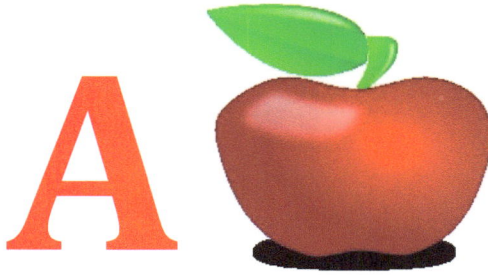

Apples!

This fruit is not only delicious, but it offers a lot of nutritional value as well. Eating apples regularly can aide in the prevention of illnesses. Like the old saying goes, "An apple a day, keeps the doctor away!" Now, whether that's true or not, I'm not exactly sure, but, it is a healthier option to choose.

Daily activity:

Round up the crew, lay flat on your back, knees bent, and let's do some sit-ups! WORK THOSE ABS!

Each person can take turns counting during each set. There's nothing to it, but to do it!

Ab workout (crunches) sets & reps: 3 sets / 12 reps

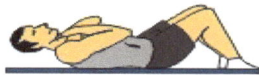

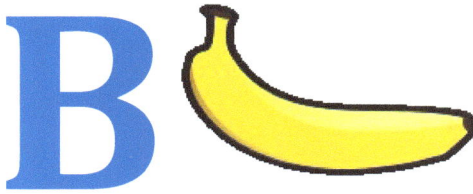

B 🍌

Bananas!

This fruit is great tasting by itself or in a bowl of cereal. Not to mention, when they're present in ice cream and milkshakes, they're to die for. ☺ Bananas contain potassium and fiber that are helpful for the digestive system.

Daily activity:

Alright, time to get up and get active!

Today's activity can be a bike ride, a game of basketball or simply going outside and tossing a ball around.

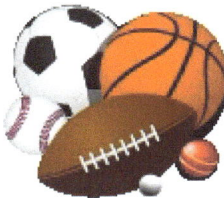

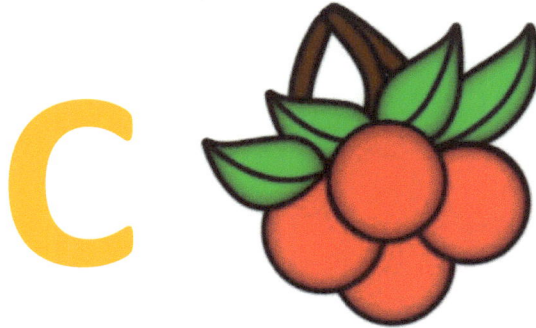

Cherries!

Loaded with vitamins and minerals, this spring time fruit is not only delicious, but has many health benefits such as, slowing or inhibiting cardiovascular, Alzheimer's and Parkinson's disease.

Daily activity:

Up on your feet! Let's go!

Calf raises (standing) 3 sets / 20 reps

(Note: You DO NOT need the barbell to do calf raises)

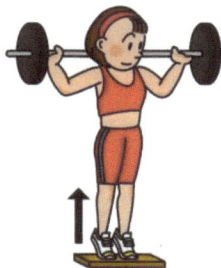

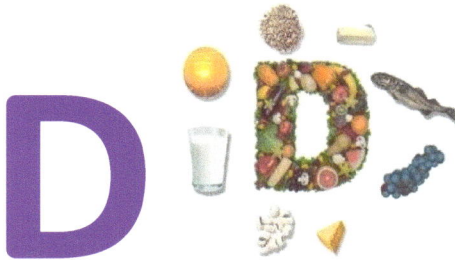

Vitamin D!

Vitamin D can be found in food sources like salmon, tuna, egg yolks, milk and cheese.

Vitamin D can also:
- help improve muscle strength
- be made by the body when exposed to ultraviolet light

Daily activity:

Alright! Turn on some music, because it's time to DANCE! Yes, dancing is a form of exercise that can help you burn large amounts of calories. So whether it's 5 minutes or 1 hour, put on your dancing shoes and dance the night away!

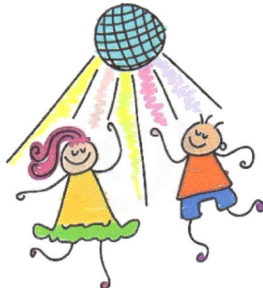

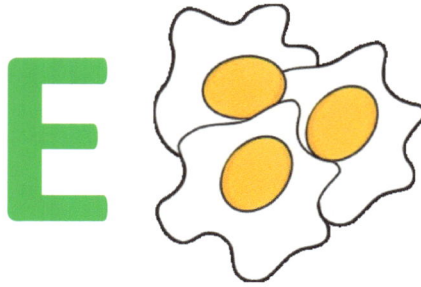

Eggs!

No breakfast would be complete without this protein packed food. Eggs are a great food full of nutrients to help you build strong muscles.

Vitamin E helps build a strong immune system, as well as healthy skin and eyes. It also plays an important role in helping prevent diseases such as Alzheimer's and diabetes.

Daily activity:

Elbows to knees 3 sets/12 reps
Lie on the floor with your hands behind your head. Curl up and touch the opposite elbow with the opposite knee. Once you do one side, that's 1 rep.

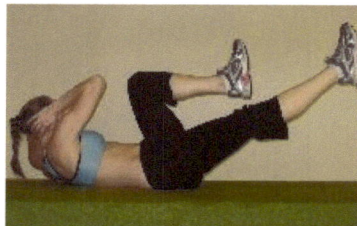

F

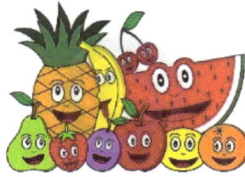

Fruits!

You were hoping I would list fries, right?! Well, NOPE! However, fruit comes in many varieties, and they all can provide essential vitamins and minerals for our daily needs. When you get hungry and are in need of a snack, fruit is a much better alternative than a candy bar, which is full of sugar and can cause bad things like:

- *Cavities*

- *Obesity*

So it is important that we make fruit a part of our daily routine. f you are in need of a snack, try eating a piece of fruit to satisfy your craving.

Daily activity:
Front lunges 3 sets/12 reps each leg

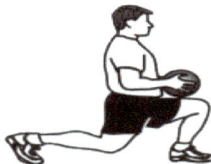

13

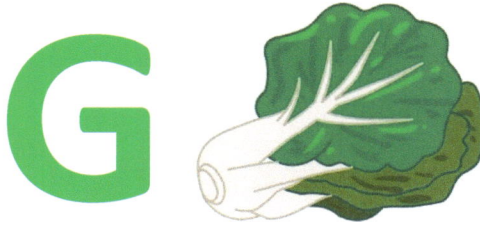

Greens!

Green vegetables are loaded with vitamins and minerals like calcium, potassium, magnesium and vitamins K, E, C and B. This food aids in providing the body with nutrients that help you to live a strong healthy life.

Adding a green vegetable to one or two meals a day can help regulate your weight and help prevent obesity.

Daily activity:
Goblet squat 3 sets / 12 reps. LET'S GO!

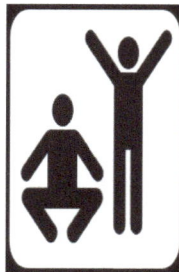

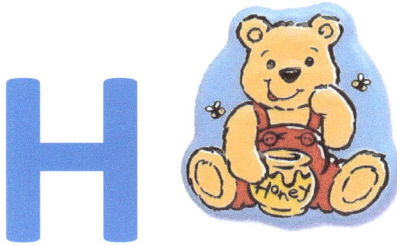

Honey!

Honey is a good substitution for sugar. You can use it to sweeten your tea, or add flavor to a meal, such as oatmeal, cream of wheat or grits. Honey also contains flavonoids, which are antioxidants that can assist with reducing the risk of some forms of cancer and heart disease.

Daily activity:
High knee jog 3 sets / 30 seconds

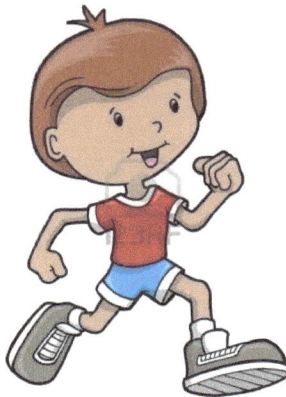

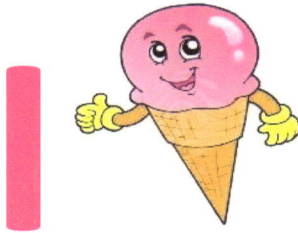

Ice cream!

Who could leave out the delicious party favorite, ice cream? Now, although ice cream is known for its high sugar content, there is a secret about ice cream that many people don't know. *Shhhhh!* Come here and I'll tell you!

Ice cream can be consumed in moderation, meaning on occasion when you've been a good boy or girl. An ice cream cone as a reward won't hurt!

Now, I know you just had this delicious treat, BUT let's still take a look at the daily activity below!

Daily Activity:
Inchworm crawl 3 sets / 12 reps

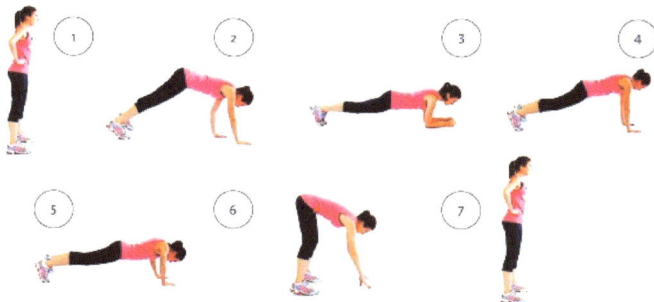

16

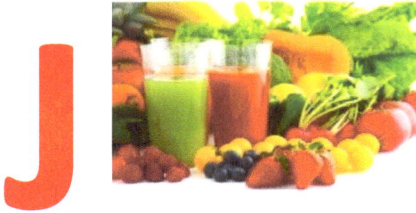

YEP, you guessed it, Juice! Now, not that really tasty, sugary, sweet kind we like, but the healthier option. Believe it or not there is one! A mixture of fresh or frozen fruits blended with some of your favorite veggies makes for a great, nutritious and delicious drink! TRY IT!

Daily Activity:
These are fun and super easy.
Jumping Jacks 3 sets / 12 reps

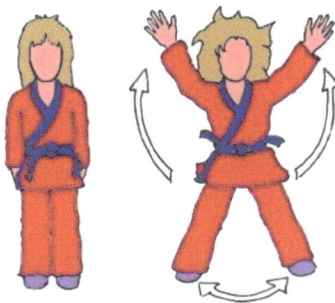

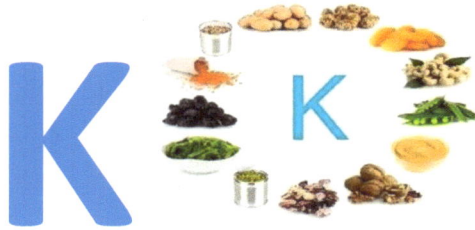

Vitamin K!

Let's throw a vitamin in here! Vitamin K aids in helping the blood clot. You know when you fall down and get a nasty cut, vitamin K can help stop the bleeding. Good sources of vitamin K come from green vegetables, beans, meat and strawberries.

Daily Activity:

Kick ball! Now this is super fun too! Grab a ball and run outside and kick it around to your friends! You'll have a blast!

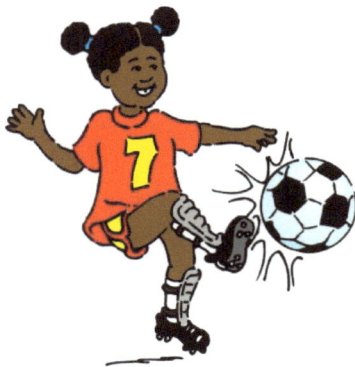

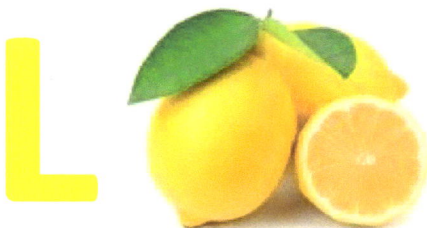

Lemons!

Lemons are one of the fruits that seem to be used in so many ways. For instance, you can make lemonade or add them to your drinking water for flavor. However, did you also know that lemons are a great source of vitamin C, vitamin B6, vitamin A, and potassium, just to name a few? It helps detox your body and your skin. Detoxing is important because it gets rid of all the nasty bugs in your body! Isn't that AWESOME?!

Daily Activity:
Lunges! 3 sets / 15 reps each leg

NOTE: You do not need any weights for this exercise.
Your body weight is just fine!

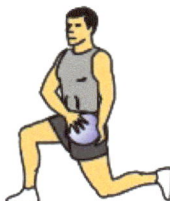

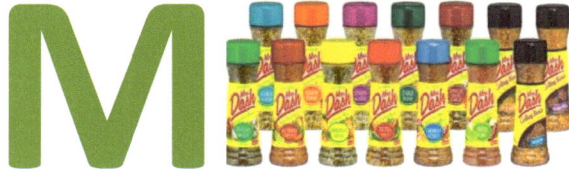

Mrs. Dash!

A huge misconception about eating healthy is that it doesn't taste good. WRONG! Mrs. Dash is a brand of seasoning that provides you with a lot of different flavors, without all the salt! Kids and adults alike can enjoy the many seasoning flavors of Mrs. Dash such as on tacos, chili, meatloaf, etc. Go ahead! Head to the store and stock up! You won't be disappointed.

Daily Activity:
Mountain climbers! Again another FUN one! Get in the push up position and take turns bringing your knees to your chest in a climbing motion! FUN right?!

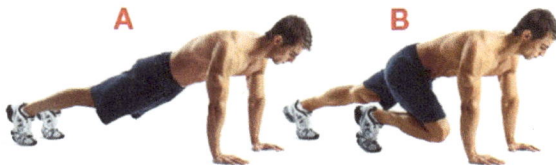

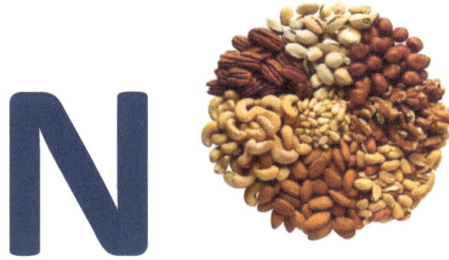

Nuts!

Yep, Nuts!! ALL kinds are a good source of protein. These are awesome healthier snack options than chips or fruit snacks. They can help you feel full even when you are hours away from eating. NO, you're not NUTs, but you should definitely eat some!

Daily Activity:
Today's daily activity is a little different. It is the word Nice! Today make someone's day by giving them a warm smile, a compliment or even playing with someone who usually plays by themselves. NICE is a word, but it can be an action too!

Go ahead try it! Now this one is super easy!

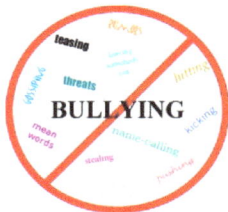
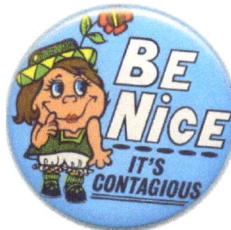

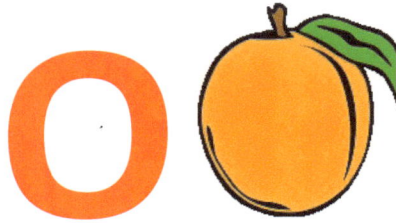

Oranges!

You can have them as a snack or as a juice at the start of your morning. Either way you'll benefit from all the nutrients contained in this fruit. It is best known for its extreme amount of vitamin C. You ever wonder why your parents or grandparents give you orange juice when you're sick, well the vitamin C helps boost your immune system! Those adults are pretty smart, huh?!

Daily Activity:
OUTDOORS! Let's just go outdoors and enjoy the weather. Take a ball or a jump rope or even some sidewalk chalk and create a great outdoors experience!

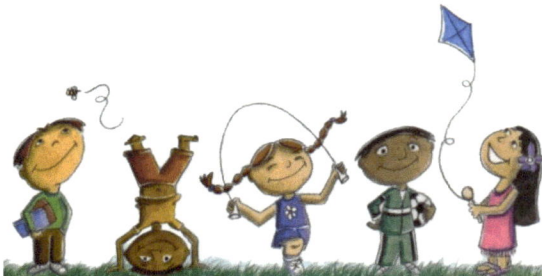

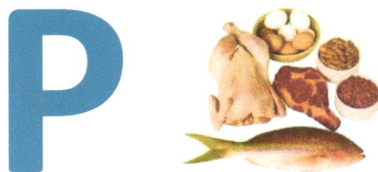

Protein!

P stands for PROTEIN, and other things as well! However, protein is the most important. It is the most valuable nutrient you can give your body. Protein can be easily obtained through milk, eggs, meats, nuts, beans, and even protein shakes! As you can see, vegetarians are also able to get this much needed nutrient by not eating any meat! Pretty cool, right?

Daily Activity:
Yep, Push Ups! Again fun, but a little more challenging. Let's see how many you can do. GO......!!

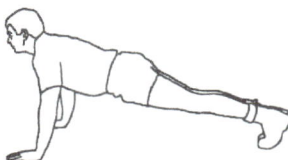

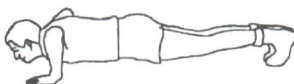

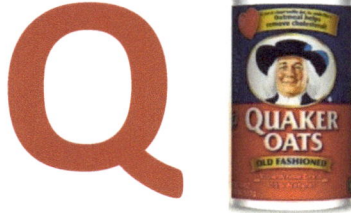

Quaker Oats!

Quaker Oats is a brand that has been around for a long time. They are best known for their variety of oatmeal flavors. They provide a great source of fiber and a great way to start off your morning. If you want to be really creative, feel free to cut up some fresh fruits and add them to your bowl of Quaker Oats! You won't regret it!

Daily Activity:
Quick Leaps 3 sets / 12 reps

Just squat like a frog and leap as fast as you can 12 times, then rest for 30 seconds and do them twice more. Ready, set, GO!

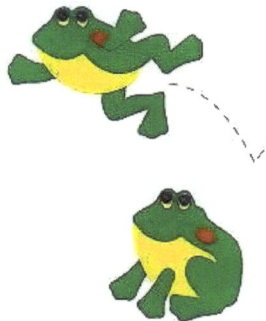

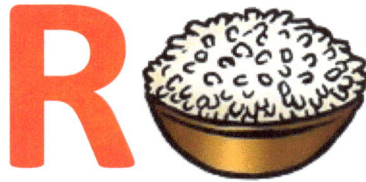

Rice!

Rice is a great addition to a lot of meals and can typically be found in many households. White rice being the most common type, can be a good source of energy if eaten an hour before or after a workout. Brown rice is also a great source for its whole grain value and its ability to provide sustained energy throughout the day. We all could use a little more energy, right?!

Daily Activity:
Running, running, and yes RUNNING! So let's get up, stretch those legs and RUN! You can run in place or go outside and RUN around!

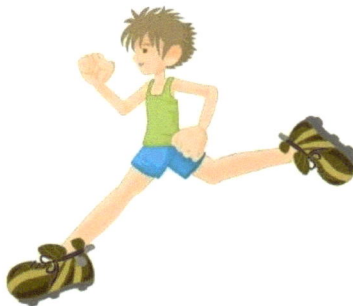

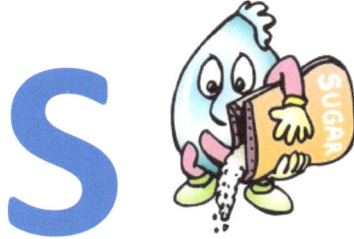

Sugar!

Sugar seems to make everything taste so much better. Our sodas, cereals, candy and so on! However, added sugar can actually do more harm than good. It can cause cavities in our teeth, as well as obesity, cardiovascular disease or diabetes. So although on the surface it seems good, sugar is not our friend and should be avoided as much as possible.

Daily Activity:
Squats are a great exercise to build strong legs and a strong core. 3 sets / 12 reps

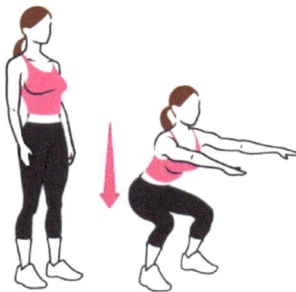

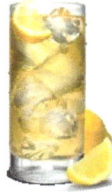

Tea!

Tea provides many great benefits for the body. Drinking tea regularly can aide in weight loss, lower cholesterol and help you to have a healthier heart. So as an alternative to soda or juice, think about having a nice glass of tea. Your body will thank you for it.

Daily Activity:
Toe Touches is today's exercise. Just lie on your back, feet in the air and reach for your toes. Let's see if we can do 3 sets 12 times.

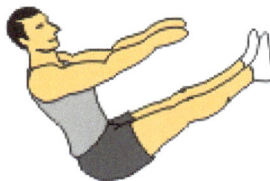

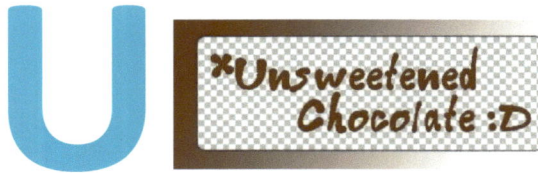

U

*Unsweetened
Chocolate :D*

Unsweetened!

Unsweetened is a label that you will see on a number of products in your local grocery store. Typically what that means is there have been no added sugars or other sweeteners to that product. However, as always, you should read the nutrition facts provided on the product to make sure there are no other hidden ingredients.

Daily Activity:
Upward Stretches is the activity for today! Stand up tall and stretch straight up - now to the right and then to the left. Let's do this for about 1 minute to loosen up our bodies.

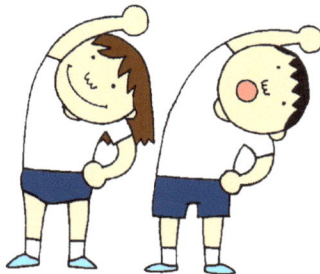

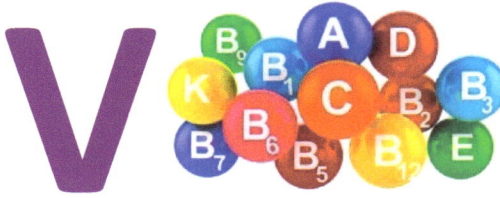

Vitamins!

Vitamins come in many forms, and they all play a key role in our daily health. Every day we should take a multi-vitamin, which contains all of the essential vitamins we need to help our bodies continue to function properly.

Daily Activity:
Vertical leaps are today's exercise. Start by getting in a squat-like position and leap straight up, then back down into the squat position. Repeat this for 3 sets, 12 repetitions.

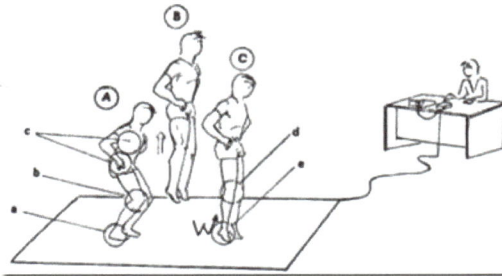

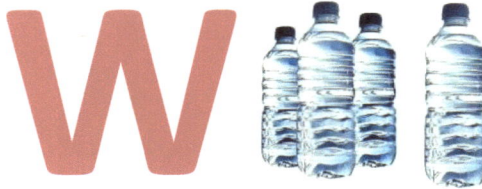

Water!

One of the most important things we need in our lives daily is water. Our bodies are made up of about 70% water. Needless to say, it is vital that we consume it daily. On average, you should have at least 8 glasses a day. Going too long without drinking water can leave your body dehydrated and with no energy. So instead of drinking a soda or juice with every meal, substitute them for a cold glass of water and truly quench your thirst.

Daily Activity:
Simply just WALK today! If you're at school, work or home, just be active today and walk a few miles. However, make sure to stay hydrated with WATER and take a buddy along with you!

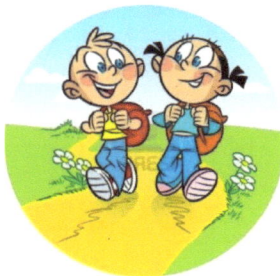

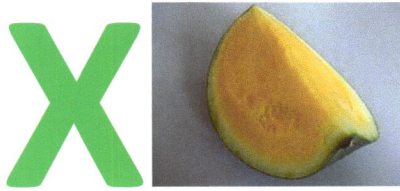

Xigua!

I know what you are thinking. … There couldn't possibly be a food that starts with the letter X. Well, actually there is and it's called Xigua. It is a form of a melon most commonly found in Africa. It is known in other countries as the watermelon. This fruit contains many nutrients, including Vitamin C and lycopene which protects our cells from damage.

Daily Activity:
Here we go - eXercise! Yeah, I know it starts with an E, but, we're exaggerating the "X". Decide what your favorite exercise is and DO IT! This is a freebie. You can do anything you want, but the important thing is to have fun while doing it. eXercising can be a great time!

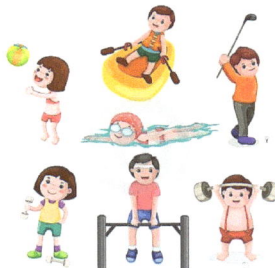

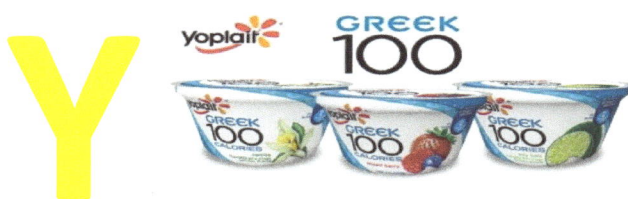

Yogurt!

Yes, Yogurt! It can be just as good as ice cream. There are plenty of different flavors to choose from as well. The Greek Yogurt brand is one of the healthier brands without all the extra sugars. Yogurt contains probiotics which is a "nice" bacterium, if you will. Probiotics help boost the immune system and can produce a healthy digestive tract. Yogurt is a dairy product, so you're getting all the nutrients you would get from milk.

Daily Activity:
Everyone can't sign up for a YOGA class today, BUT we can take on the yoga state of relaxation. So go ahead, relax today! Do something that relaxes you like coloring or reading a book or watching a movie. You worked hard up to this point so enjoy this daily activity!

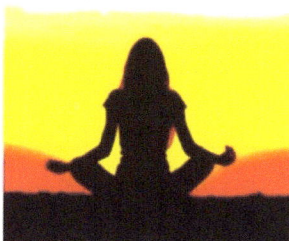

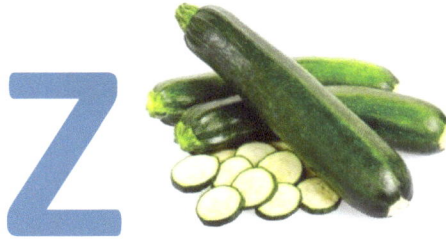

Zucchini!

You did it! You made it to Z. Now let's look at this vegetable called, Zucchini. Zucchini can serve multiple purposes. Packed with vitamin C, as well as B6 and potassium, zucchini can be eaten in a variety of ways. There is zucchini bread. It can be made into pasta, and it can simply be cut up and eaten raw. This particular veggie also has high water content and is great for hydrating yourself.

Daily Activity:
No, we can't go zip – lining! But we can create our own Zumba class wherever we are. Go ahead and try it! Turn on some salsa music or just something upbeat and create your own dance steps. Time to move, move, move!

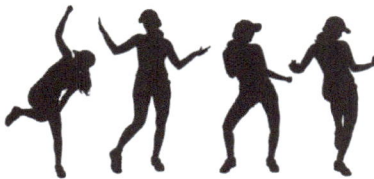

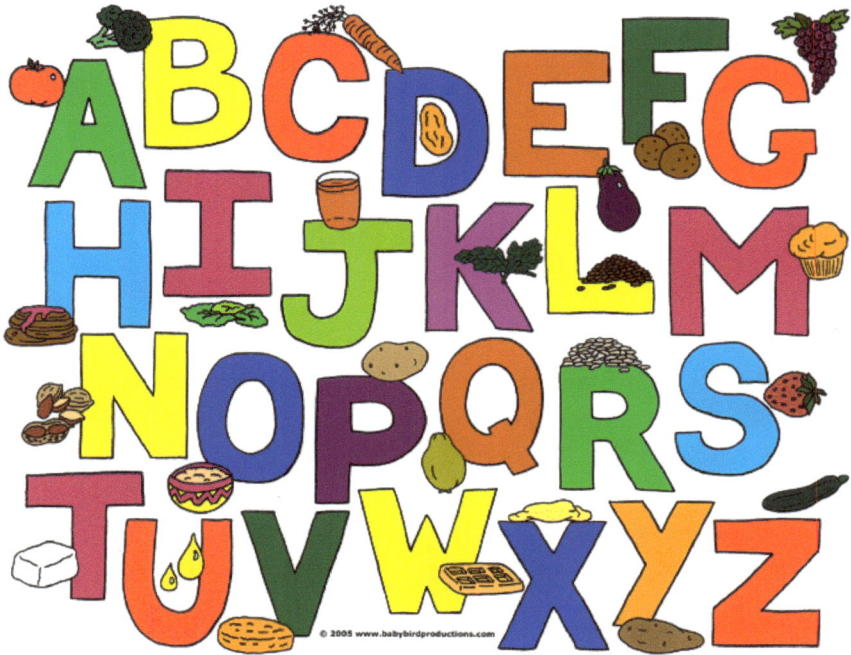

CONGRATULATIONS!

You have completed the *ABCs* to health and wellness! I hope you've enjoyed learning your alphabet. Remember these tips, and daily activities can be repeated as often as you like. You can even grab a new partner the next time around!

ABOUT THE AUTHORS

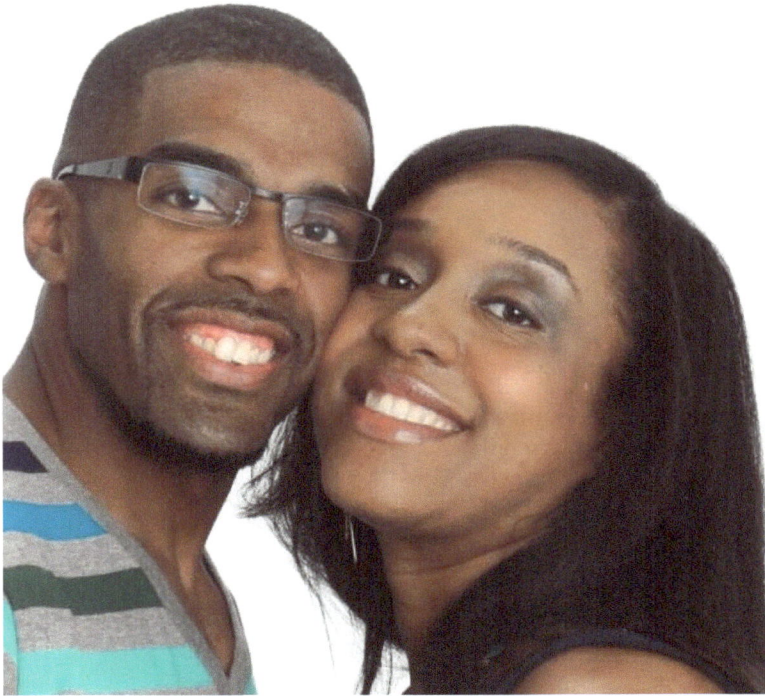

Arian and Megan Smith

Arian Smith, founder and CEO of A-Z Fitness, began this fitness journey over 15 years ago. Now as an ISSA Certified Fitness Trainer and Sports Nutrition Specialist, he has lent his knowledge, skills and most of all his passion for healthier living, to the world. He embarked on the book journey after realizing that there was a crowd we still needed to tap into, and that was our children. It wasn't all about competing in fitness shows and winning anymore. It was bigger than that! With two young children of his own, they became the reason for a healthier lifestyle. He hopes that this book will reach families, schools, churches, youth camps and any other place where a young life is evolving. That the content will help in the journey to healthier living.

Megan Smith, MBA in Health Services Management, co-founder and CFO of A-Z Fitness, jumped on board right alongside her husband with the passion and drive to see people succeed in their health goals. Working in the healthcare environment for over 8 years and seeing the various illness and conditions that people suffered with (both young and old), gave her a different view on healthier living. Never having weighed over 160 lbs. (unless with child), she was still not healthy. She learned with the help of her husband that this has to be a lifestyle, and they have to be there for their girls. With the same hope as Arian, Megan wants to see this book reach the masses and do what it was designed to do and that's help you in your fitness and health walk.

Dedicated to Kyndall and Leeya Smith
Mommy and Daddy love you!

www.ingramcontent.com/pod-product-compliance
Lightning Source LLC
Chambersburg PA
CBHW041223270326
41933CB00001B/24